THE ESSENTIAL GUIDE TO

Natural Pet Care

EPILEPSY

THE ESSENTIAL GUIDE TO

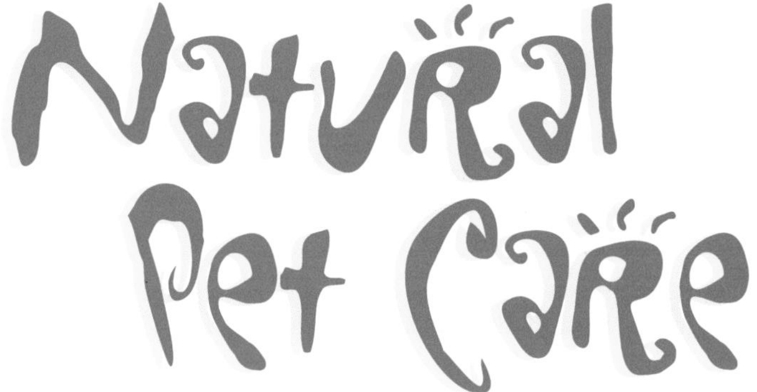

EPILEPSY

CAL OREY

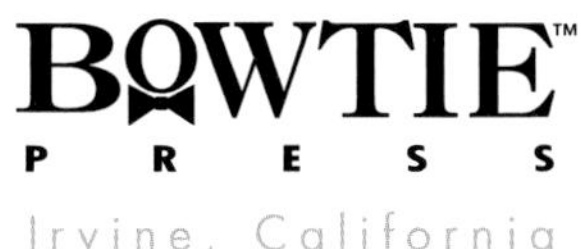

Irvine, California

Thanks to the Redwood City Library, Redwood City, California, and
the San Carlos Library, San Carlos, California. —C.O.

Ruth Berman, editor-in-chief
Nick Clemente, special consultant
Book design and layout by Michele Lanci-Altomare and Victor W. Perry
Mike Uyesugi, cover design

Library of Congress Cataloging-in-Publication Data

Orey, Cal, 1952-
Epilepsy / Cal Orey.
p. cm. -- (The essential guide to natural pet care)
Includes bibliographical references (p.).
ISBN 1-889540-34-X (pbk. : alk. paper)
1. Dogs--Diseases. 2. Cats--Diseases. 3.Epilepsy in animals.
I. Title. II. Series.
SF992.E57074 1998
636.7'0896853--dc21 98-39298
CIP

BowTie™ Press
3 Burroughs
Irvine, California 92618

Manufactured in the United States of America
10 9 8 7 6 5 4 3 2 1

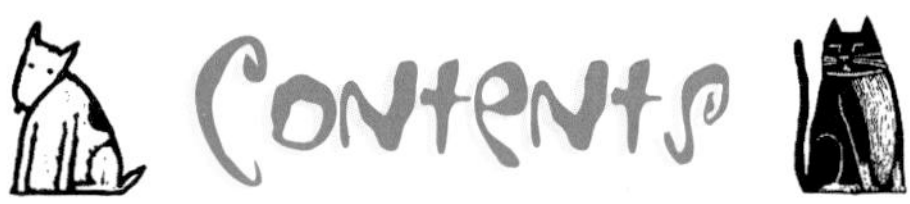

FOREWORD

Complementary medicine (also known as holistic or alternative medicine) has become increasingly popular as an addition to or sometimes even a replacement for conventional medicine. Conventional medicine concentrates on getting immediate results using substances to control a disease process or replace something that is missing. It is invaluable in situations where fast action is imperative, such as severe shock or where surgery is needed to save a life. Conventional medicine also has diagnostic tools that help us better understand what is going on in the body.

When there is a long-standing problem, when the side effects of conventional medicine are almost as bad as the disease, or when the body isn't functioning quite like it should, holistic medicine often offers a better solution. The approach in holistic medicine is to help the body heal itself with a minimum of side effects. When used to complement conventional medicine, holistic, or complementary, medicine can speed up healing time, decrease side effects, or increase survival time in chronic diseases.

Not everyone is patient enough to appreciate complementary medicine. Some of my clients are unwilling to wait the month or more that some methods take to work. Practitioners of conventional medicine may look askance on the jargon or ideas associated with holistic medicine. Those who are accustomed to using a single drug to treat a single problem distrust the multiple chemicals present in one herb, or the multiple herbs in a Chinese formula. Others distrust anything originating in a Third World country. These are problems of philosophy and perception, not problems of effectiveness of the procedure.

Many veterinarians are unable to find research about holistic methods. There is a growing body of research in support of complementary medicine, but it is scattered, and much of it is found in obscure journals and in languages other than English. There is no easy way to find research in complementary medicine. The research often uses clinical studies, not the "gold standard" double-blind study favorite of the medical profession.

In a double-blind study, a single drug is tested, and neither the practitioner nor the owner knows whether the pet is getting the actual treatment or a placebo. In complementary medicine, the treatment encompasses diet, supplements, physical treatment, herbs, homeopathy, etc. Each holistic method contributes a separate effect and works best when combined with other methods; there is no single active ingredient to the treatment. Studies of only one method often show poor results. With hands-on treatments such as acupuncture, the practitioner always knows whether or not the treatment is real, so double-blind studies are impossible. Clinical tests comparing the results from using holistic therapy with the results from using conventional medicine show that holistic medicine usually equals or surpasses conventional medicine.

Holistic professional journals and associations share this information and filter out the unproven. The medical backgrounds of the professionals behind these journals and associations help them evaluate the evidence, and their holistic backgrounds teach them not to reject things too quickly. Books such as this one with in-depth research that is cross-checked with a holistic practitioner are the best way for pet owners like you to become informed.

—Nancy Scanlan, D.V.M.

What Is Epilepsy?

In a rustic bungalow in San Carlos, California, at 4:00 in the afternoon, an orange-and-white Brittany spaniel named Dylan grows restless; he cowers and soon flees toward the backdoor. Suddenly, his body stiffens and falls over. All four legs stick out, rigid. Within seconds, Dylan loses consciousness and jerks violently.

The episode subsides in less than three minutes, but the owner feels as if the frightening event lasts for an eternity.

Dylan has just experienced a seizure.

One hour later, he chews his bone as if nothing had happened out of the ordinary. But it had.

One of the most upsetting experiences for a pet owner is to watch his or her pet having a seizure. But the fact is, seizures in companion animals are a more common phenomenon than many people realize. Experts estimate that the overall incidence of seizure disorders in dogs and cats occur in 1 percent of these species.

Because the seizures that Dylan had after his first one were infrequent and less intense, his owner had two options. She could give her four-legged companion anticonvulsant drugs that might help him, but all drugs have side effects. Or she could opt for alternative therapies to control epilepsy naturally. She chose to use natural therapies.

Epilepsy is not a single disease. It is repeated, intermittent seizures with an unknown cause. Seizures, also called convulsions or fits, are caused by any process that alters normal brain function. "When neurons that fire electrical impulses in the brain go haywire, they short-circuit normal brain processes, resulting in a seizure," explains Stephen Blake, D.V.M., a veterinarian with a holistic consultation practice in San Diego, California.

Seizures can occur in dogs and cats of all ages, according to experts, and can be caused by two major groups of problems: brain problems and nonbrain problems. Brain problems that may cause seizures include true epilepsy (also known as idiopathic epilepsy—a form of seizure that usually begins between six months and two years of age); brain infections (viral, bacterial, fungal, and protozoal); degenerative conditions of the brain tissue; hydrocephalus (water on the brain); brain tumors; stroke-like conditions; blood clots in the brain; and an injury to the head. Nonbrain problems that may cause seizures include ingested poisons, kidney disease, liver disease, heart disease, low blood sugar, nerve and muscle problems, and infections.

The origin of the epileptic condition falls into two categories: idiopathic or acquired. Idiopathic (without a known cause) epilepsy is genetic, or hereditary. Acquired epilepsy is usually caused by an outside source (such as toxins, infective organisms, and trauma). Other sources include nutritional deficiencies, metabolic disorders, and tumors.

At Ohio State University, one study of fifty healthy dogs who had suffered one or more seizures suggests that seizures that happen more than once a month may be a sign of a developmental, metabolic, or infectious process. Neither the sex of the dog nor whether or not the dog is neutered makes a difference in predicting the cause of the seizures.

Additionally, experts claim that seizures in a dog younger than one year old are often due to congenital or genetic problems, infections, or toxins. Dogs between one and five years of age (and as young as six months) who are normal between epileptic fits, such as Dylan, often have idiopathic epilepsy. A dog older than six is likely to have tumors or infectious or inflammatory problems that are causing the seizures.

Ongoing studies prove that the origin of epilepsy, for the most part, is the same for humans as it is for dogs. With some breeds of dogs, it's genetic. Cats, on the other hand, have an underlying acquired cause for their seizures, says Karen Vernau, D.V.M., a neurology resident at the UC Davis Veterinary School of Medicine. And author Richard Pitcairn, D.V.M., Ph.D., says, "Although epilepsy is fairly common in dogs, it is rather unusual in cats."

Common causes of feline seizures include poisoning; head injury from being hit by a car, which may cause delayed seizures; feline leukemia virus (FeLV), feline infectious peritonitis (FIP); fungal infection; chemical toxins; brain tumors; heatstroke; liver dysfunction; and renal failure. To uncover the cause of a feline seizure, says Dr. Vernau, a complete cell count, serum biochemistry profile, urinalysis, and FeLV antigen test are required. Plus, other tests from electroencephalograms (EEG), which trace brain waves, to cranial CAT (computerized axial tomography) scans or MRIs (magnetic resonance imaging) may also help determine the underlying cause. Dr. Scanlan suggests also testing for feline immunodeficiency virus (FIV) and feline infectious peritonitis (FIP).

Sometimes cats are born with a brain disorder that causes seizures. As with dogs, idiopathic epilepsy in cats is likely to strike between six months and three years of age.

And although epilepsy is rare in horses, it does appear in cattle (Brown Swiss and Swedish red). As of yet, no conclusive studies have determined whether other animals such as birds, reptiles, or rabbits are prone to epilepsy.

Dog breeders should beware: Current research shows epilepsy is found not just in all purebreds but in mixed breeds as well. The Belgian Tervuren is listed among the breeds in which a genetic factor plays a role. Other breeds highly suspected of being prone to epilepsy include the beagle, cocker spaniel, collie, dachshund, German shepherd, golden retriever, Irish setter, keeshond, Labrador retriever, Saint Bernard, Siberian husky, wire-haired terrier, all poodles, and all schnauzers.

Epilepsy in purebred dogs is becoming the focus of more and more research and for good reason. Breeding studies show that when both sire and dam are epileptic or when an accidental mating of two related epileptic dogs happens, epileptic puppies are often the result.

In addition, experts report that in purebred dogs, the incidence of seizure disorders may be 15 to 20 percent because of the presence of inherited (idiopathic) epilepsy in those breeds. The bottom line is that no epileptic dog should be bred. That means without exception female dogs with epilepsy should be spayed and male dogs should be neutered.

TREATING EPILEPSY HOLISTICALLY

The ultimate goal of alternative animal medicine, according to holistic practitioners, is to train the animal's body to fix itself. "Alternative treatments are based on the belief that our pets' bodies know what to do to heal themselves," says Dr. Blake. "Conventional drug therapies don't work *with* the body to produce the healing process."

"Control with drugs suppresses the brain function," adds Dr. Pitcairn. "We use alternative healthy therapies for pets to cure the condition so the seizures don't happen anymore." Many pet owners, however, are not aware that techniques such as diet therapy, homeopathy, herbology, and acupuncture can be a godsend to the health and well-being of their epileptic pets.

Take Carolyn Ball, for instance. She owns an epileptic American Eskimo dog and is desperately seeking help. "Angel is aptly named. She is a sweet-natured socialite, snow-white and beautiful. At eight months she had her first seizure. We were so frightened.... It lasted forty seconds. Afterward, she continued to lay there and quiver for two to three hours. We took her to the emergency room.

They kept her overnight and said that it may never happen again," she says.

But it has. Since the first seizure, Angel has had about forty seizures, one occurring about every three weeks. Meanwhile, the young dog is on phenobarbital. But the seizures lately have been episodic over a twenty-four-hour period. Carolyn doesn't know whom to turn to for help.

Can natural options help Angel and countless other dogs and cats with seizure disorders? Absolutely, say holistic experts.

Less severe forms of epilepsy can be treated wholly with alternative methods; however, the worst forms of epilepsy are currently being treated with a combination of conventional and alternative methods, according to Dr. Scanlan. Conventional drugs, such as the anticonvulsants phenobarbital, primidone, diazepam (Valium), and potassium bromide, are often used in these cases.

Phenobarbital is currently considered the drug of choice; long-term use, however, can destroy liver cells. When the drug is stopped suddenly, signs of physical withdrawal can include tremors, restlessness, and the return of seizures.

Primidone is often used in dogs, but it doesn't seem to help cats, and it also can cause liver damage. Diazepam is effective only in bringing a pet out of ongoing convulsions. And the side effects of potassium bromide can include stomach irritation or nausea. All anticonvulsants can cause decreased alertness, varying from lethargy to stupor.

When medications are combined with natural therapies, the dosage of medications often can be reduced after a few months if seizures occur less frequently. And remember that holistic treatments can and do play a lifelong role in maintaining a healthier pet while controlling epilepsy naturally.

CHAPTER 1

Recognizing Epilepsy

WHAT ARE THE WARNING SIGNS AND SYMPTOMS?

Being able to pinpoint the telltale signals of a seizure may be one of the best things you can do for your epileptic pet's health. This ability will put you on top of an untimely seizure attack if one happens to your dog, cat, or any furry friend.

There are two basic types of seizures: petit mal and grand mal. Infrequent petit mal seizures are brief fits, usually involving nodding, chewing, licking, or minor

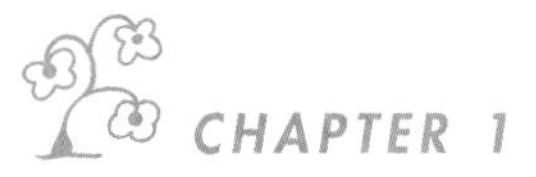

twitching. Dogs often collapse into a sitting or lying position but don't fall over on their sides. They tend to have a partial loss of consciousness with a faraway look in their eyes. The frequently occurring grand mal seizures are more severe. Cats are more apt to experience grand mal than petit mal seizures. Grand mal, or major motor seizures, include a loss of consciousness and large body movements.

There are three stages of a grand mal seizure: the aura, the ictus, and the postictus.

The aura stage signals the beginning of the seizure. The animal may pace, whine, tremble, be affectionate, wander, hide, or flee. The aura may last a few seconds or many hours before the actual seizure begins, and it can alert owners that a seizure is imminent.

The ictus is the seizure, characterized by sudden stiffening and shaking of all the muscle groups, followed by running movements. It usually lasts one to three minutes.

The postictus follows the seizure. The animal may be confused, restless, unresponsive, excited, panting heavily, or may want to go outside.

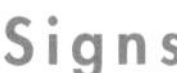

Signs

The aura can be even more frightening than the seizure itself because it's like getting a hurricane or tornado warning. Your cat acting as if "invisible aliens" are following her, or your dog darting under a table in fear is a scary prediction to what's ahead.

Dylan's owner remembers one day a few years ago when her energetic sporting dog appeared more active than normal. The dog owner had no clue that it was a probable precursor to a "big one" (a grand mal seizure). Later that day, Dylan cowered and then made a quick dash into the bathroom for refuge. It was as if an earthquake had hit.

Not all epileptic pets experience the aura. And not all pet owners experience the warning. Just ask Joan Hostetler. "I've had my epileptic Welsh corgi, Rusty, age two and a half, for only three months. So far I've not been able to see a pattern before he has a seizure. My other animals (a dog and a cat) don't sense it as some animals do. Rusty has most of his seizures at night or while he is sleeping on the couch. Once, I could hear him walking across the kitchen floor, and he suddenly fell over with a thud," she says.

"He shakes quite violently for thirty seconds to one minute. His teeth chatter, he foams at the mouth, and he urinates. He apparently is blind—or at least unaware of his surroundings—for three or four minutes, then he becomes very thirsty and hungry. Within ten minutes he is back to normal as if nothing has happened," Hostetler recalls.

Symptoms

What are the most common seizure symptoms? The pet stiffens, usually loses consciousness, urinates and salivates involuntarily, jerks intermittently and paddles, and then recovers. The seizure may last one to five minutes. Afterward, the animal may seem exhausted, confused, and disoriented for minutes or hours. And most likely the pet's owner is dazed even longer.

Besides petit mal and grand mal seizures, other types exist as well:

- Partial seizures (focal seizures): Movements are restricted to one area of the body, such as muscle jerking, movement of one limb, or facial twitching.

- Complex partial seizures (psychomotor seizures): These are linked with bizarre behaviors such as fly biting (snapping at the air as if the dog were snapping at flies), hysterical running, cowering, or hiding. Vomiting, diarrhea, abdominal distress, salivation, and temporary blindness are other signs.

Cluster seizures: These are multiple seizures that occur within a short span of time with only brief periods of consciousness.

Status epilepticus: Status epilepticus can happen as one continuous seizure lasting thirty minutes or more or as a series of multiple seizures in a short time with no periods of normal consciousness. It can end in death if not controlled.

HOW TO TELL IF YOUR PET HAS EPILEPSY

Welcome to the world of multiple causes for seizures, which makes diagnosis of any pet difficult and frustrating. The fact remains that "epilepsy is a diagnosis dilemma that is usually made only after other possibilities—such as worms, poisons, low blood sugar, and tumors—have been ruled out. Thus, it is sort of diagnosis by default, and the epilepsy may actually be caused by a mixed bag of things," says Dr. Pitcairn.

Of course, one seizure is not a diagnosis but a potential sign of an underlying problem. After one fit, it is difficult to predict if your pet will have another seizure or not, but a complete history and physical exam will help provide your doctor with vital information.

"If the seizures happen infrequently and are quite mild, your veterinarian may simply advise you to observe the condition and to report back if the seizures increase in severity or frequency," says Bob Goldstein, V.M.D.

The usual recommended tests are urinalysis, complete blood count and blood chemistry, fasting blood glucose level, serum glucose level, serum lead level, and fecal parasite or ova examination. Additional tests may include a CAT scan or MRI, spinal fluid tap (CSF), and an EEG. The purpose of these tests is to tell whether the problem stems from the brain or from other parts of the body, since the prognosis and kinds of treatment differ for diseases stemming from these areas.

Still, not one test for epilepsy in the dog or cat exists; even the EEG is not a perfect epilepsy detector. The good news is that once epilepsy has been diagnosed, a pet owner has options for treatment.

CHAPTER 2

Antiseizure Natural Remedies

There are many natural remedies for treating epilepsy. Is one any better than the others? That's hard to say. Here is a look at seven options. You'll discover the holistic method that works best for your pet and learn how to control epilepsy in the process. Be sure to consult with a veterinarian who is knowledgeable in the field before beginning any type of treatment or dietary change.

REMEDY #1
ACUPUNCTURE

Acupuncture involves the insertion

of fine needles into specific points on the body. There are more than three hundred points, but most veterinarians regularly use only about one hundred and generally just six to twenty at a time. These needles stimulate nerve fibers that induce the body to release pain-relieving endorphins, those feel-good hormones. Some veterinarians find this ancient Chinese therapy to be the most effective holistic treatment for epilepsy. "It has a record of greatly decreasing or even stopping epilepsy," says Dr. Scanlan.

Sometimes gold beads are implanted in the acupuncture sites for extended stimulation. Gold bead implants consist of pin-size pure gold, gold-plated, or gold wire pieces that are inserted under the skin. They are available from Chinese medical suppliers. Dr. Jeffrey Bryan, a San Francisco–area veterinarian, explains how they work, "The gold beads are implanted in the acupuncture sites, where you want extended stimulation for up to a period of one year. They're used for pain relief, particularly around the joints, and they can also be used for seizure control."

Buffy is one dog who has benefited from acupuncture. A nine-year-old Pomeranian, Buffy used to suffer frequent grand mal seizures. Initially, drug therapy (oral phenobarbital) seemed to offer some control, but Buffy's owner decided to seek holistic treatment as well. Buffy's holistic veterinarian recommended acupuncture treatments on a regular basis (about once every two months).

After just a few treatments, Buffy's seizures decreased, and then the people-loving canine became seizure-free for two years.

"Acupuncture is not usually considered a substitute for drug therapy but is used in conjunction with it. Of five dogs with intractable epilepsy who were treated with gold bead implants in acupuncture points, only two dogs relapsed after five months. Two reports of epileptic dogs given acupuncture in the ear (Shen-men-point) are more positive. One dog enjoyed a sixfold increase in time between seizures; the other was seizure-free for two hundred days after a previous history of monthly seizures," reports Alicia Wiersma-Aylward, author of *Canine Epilepsy*.

To find a certified veterinary acupuncturist in your area, contact the International Veterinary Acupuncture Society by sending a SASE in care of IVAS, P.O. Box 1478, Longmont, CO 80502.

REMEDY #2
A NATURAL DIET

Holistic practitioners recommend feeding an epileptic pet a home-prepared diet of fresh food that excludes all commercial foods, snacks, or foods containing additives or coloring agents. "Nutrition should be geared toward preventing the intake of substances that may irritate the brain tissue," reports Dr. Pitcairn. "Chemicals in the pet's diet can aggravate an underlying inflammatory condition in the brain, which is why animals are prone to seizures," he explains.

Dr. Pitcairn also suggests a vegetarian diet for an epileptic pet. "Many human epileptics are significantly helped by avoiding meat," he explains, "and it may help pets as well." Dr. Pitcairn suggests feeding your pet a vegetarian diet for at least three months to see if it helps. For cats, consider low-meat recipes, rather than a completely vegetarian diet. (Recipes follow at end of remedy.)

Alfred J. Plechner, D.V.M., says, "food allergies should always be suspected. In my practice I always recommend that an epileptic animal be placed on a low-protein hypoallergenic diet." Hypoallergenic pet food often consists of chicken and rice, fish and rice, or soy-based products (such as tofu) and rice. This diet creates the least amount of allergies for the cat or dog.

Dr. Plechner recalls a colleague, Dr. Wilson, who was baffled by one patient, a three-year-old female golden retriever. The canine suffered uncontrollable epilepsy in spite of primadone therapy. "We talked by phone about the case, and I suggested feeding her a nonmeat kibble. The new diet was started and no new seizures occurred.

This encouraged Dr. Wilson to start weaning the dog slowly off the medication." The dog stayed on a hypoallergenic diet, and the seizures stopped. The dog is now drug-free. "Here was an animal unable to be controlled by any drug and who was certain to be put to sleep. By treating the cause, instead of the end result, the suffering stopped and the dog's life was saved," explains Dr. Plechner.

After Dr. Plechner began a private veterinary practice in Hollywood, CA, one of his early patients, a cat named Oscar, fell victim to grand mal seizures and was kept sedated for years on phenobarbital. The owner was feeding him a diet of canned and dry food. "I suggested she try cooking a rice and chicken combination for the cat to see if that might help. The seizures quickly stopped, and we were able to reduce the phenobarbital and then cut it out altogether. The cat did fine afterward. Something in the commercial diet was causing the epilepsy," recalls Dr. Plechner.

Both Oscar and the golden retriever are good illustrations of how pets are benefiting from pet owners and veterinarians who are learning that nutrition may be a key to controlling seizures.

You can make your own home-prepared meals for your epileptic pet with ingredients from a supermarket or health food store. To help you get started, here are a few holistic veterinarians' healthful recipes:

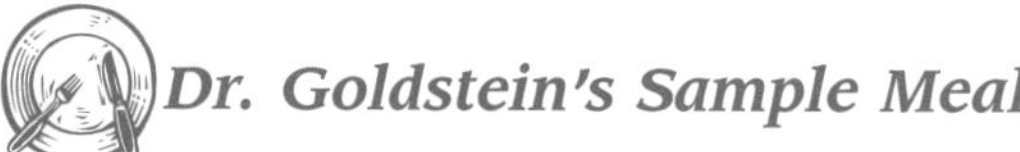

Dr. Goldstein's Sample Meal

	35-lb Dog	10-lb Cat
**Natural base food (dry)*	*½ cup*	*¼ cup*
Brown rice, cooked	*¼ cup*	*⅛ cup*
Organic carrots, grated	*¼ cup*	*⅛ cup*
Sesame oil	*2 tsp*	*½ tsp*
Organic garlic	*1 clove*	*½ clove*
Organic low-fat yogurt	*2 tsp*	*1 tsp*
*** Cooked meat or chicken*	*¼ cup*	*⅛ cup*

Adjust quantities according to your pet's weight. Mix ingredients together and serve an entire meal twice a day.

** Natural commercial foods that Dr. Goldstein recommends are California Natural; Cornucopia; Lick Your Chops; Natural Life; Nature's Recipe; Nutro's Natural Choice; Precise; Pet Guard Premium; Sojouner Farms Natural Dog Food; Solid Gold Hund-N-Flocken; and Wysong.*

*** Occasionally you can feed your pet extra meat, preferably from a source that's free of hormones and antibiotics.*

Dr. Goldstein's Favorite Healthy Snacks

Apple, chopped

Brussels sprout

Homemade popcorn

Melon ball

Organic applesauce

Organic banana

Organic grape

Pear, chopped

Sugar-Free Shredded Wheat

Whole carrot

Whole wheat matzo

Zucchini stick

Feed a 10-lb animal one treat, the portion about the size of a grape, once a day; adjust quantities based on your own pet's weight. A pet who has a stable and healthy weight can have more. If your pet is at all overweight, stick to the recommended dosage of one grape-size piece per day for a 10-lb animal.

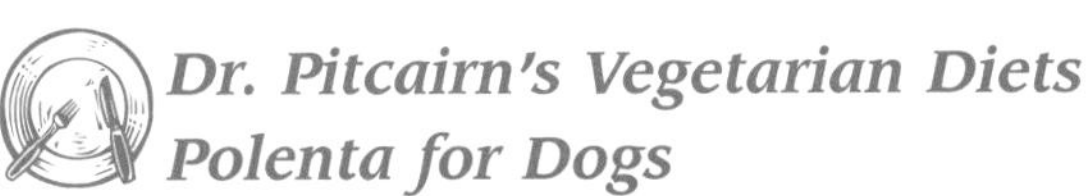

Dr. Pitcairn's Vegetarian Diets Polenta for Dogs

½ cup powdered milk + 4 cups water (or 4 cups low-fat milk)

1 cup cornmeal

2 eggs, beaten

2½ cups grated cheese

600 milligrams (mg) calcium (or ½ tsp eggshell powder or 1 tsp bonemeal)

1 Tbs Healthy Powder (see recipe p.16)

1 tsp vegetable oil
100–200 IU vitamin E
15 mg iron supplement
½ cup vegetables (optional)

Bring powdered milk and water to a boil. (If using low-fat milk instead of powder and water, scald and stir to avoid burning.) Add the cornmeal quickly with a whisk and blend until smooth. Cover and reduce heat to simmer until the cornmeal is soft and mushy, about 10 minutes. While the cornmeal is still hot, blend in the eggs and cheese. After some cooling, stir in the remaining ingredients. Divide the total quantity in half and feed one half in the morning and one half in the evening. (Large dogs are less likely to bloat when fed twice a day.)

Substitutes for the cornmeal: 1 cup millet (+ 3 cups water = 3 cups cooked); 1 cup whole wheat couscous (+ 1½ cups water = 2½ cups cooked); 2 cups raw oats (+ 4 cups water = 4 cups oatmeal).

Yield: About 5½ cups with 210 kilocalories per cup.

Daily ration: toy—⅔ to 2½ cups; small—2½ to 5 cups; medium—5 to 6½ cups; large—6½ to 9 cups; giant—9 to 13½ cups+.

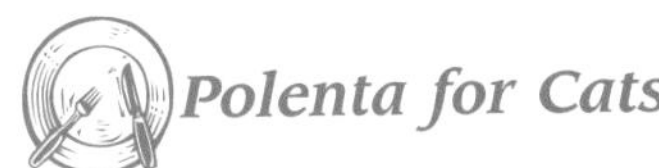

Polenta for Cats

½ cup cornmeal or polenta (or about 2 cups cooked)

4 eggs, beaten

½ cup grated cheese

1 Tbs Healthy Powder (see recipe p.16)

2 Tbs nutritional yeast

1,000 mg calcium
(or rounded ½ tsp eggshell powder or 1¾ tsp bonemeal)

50–100 IU vitamin E

200 mg taurine supplement (found in many cat vitamins)

1–2 tsp protein powder—from lactalbumin or egg albumin (optional)

1 tsp vegetables with each meal (optional)

Bring 2 cups of water to a boil. Add the cornmeal or polenta, stirring briskly with a fork or whisk. (Or mix the meal in ½ cup cold water first and add this to 1½ cups boiling water.) When blended, cover and simmer about 10 minutes or until the cornmeal is a smooth mush. While it is still hot, stir in the eggs and cheese. After the mixture has cooled, stir in the remaining ingredients. (Heat can destroy taurine.)

Substitutes for corn or polenta: ½ cup millet (+ 1½ cups water = 1½ cups cooked); ½ cup whole wheat couscous (+ ¾ cup water = 1¼ cups cooked); or 1 cup raw oats (+ 2 cups water = 2 cups oatmeal).

Yield: About 3¾ cups, with about 240 kilocalories per cup. Feed 1 to 1½ cups a day—more if your cat is active.

"This recipe derives 71 percent of its protein from meatless animal sources, so be sure to add the taurine," advises Dr. Pitcairn.

Healthy Powder

2 cups nutritional (torula) yeast

1 cup lecithin granules

¼ cup kelp powder

¼ cup bonemeal (or 9,000 mg calcium or 5 tsp eggshell powder)

1,000 mg vitamin C (ground) or ¼ tsp sodium ascorbate (optional)

Mix all ingredients together in a 1-quart container and refrigerate.

Add to each recipe as instructed. You may also add this mixture to commercial food as follows: 1 to 2 tsp per day for cats or small dogs; 2 to 3 tsp per day for medium-size dogs; 1 to 2 Tbs per day for large dogs.

(*From* Dr. Pitcairn's Complete Guide to Natural Health for Dogs and Cats)

REMEDY #3
FAT INTAKE

Veterinarians recommend feeding epileptic pets a high-fat diet. "The increased fat in the blood decreases the excitability of the neurons in the brain," reports Dr. Scanlan. "In response, this stops seizures by changing brain chemistry. A high-fat diet that includes Omega-3 and Omega-6 fatty acids (not all do), can help decrease inflammation of the brain."

One example of a high-fat diet is the ketogenic diet (k-diet), although it is still experimental. Many human epileptics have been helped by eating the k-diet, which may help pets as well. So if no other diet seems to work for your pet, the ketogenic diet may be the one that finally does the trick. [For k-diet guidelines, see pp. 34–35] "If you're interested in a ketogenic diet for your pet, first consult with your vet to make sure it gets enough of the nutrients, such as lecithin and choline, that are involved in processing fat," suggests Dr. Scanlan. "In an undernourished body, the sheath insulating the nerves thins because the body doesn't have the nutrients to regenerate this protective tissue. Lecithin is one of the nutrients essential to making that sheath," says Dr. Goldstein. Dr. Scanlan warns to make sure that your pet doesn't have a condition such as diabetes or pancreatitis that can become worse on a k-diet.

To get a rich source of lecithin for your pet, along with other essential vitamins and minerals, use a product such as Daily Health Nuggets. Contact Earth Animal at 1-800-711-2292.

REMEDY #4
ANTIOXIDANTS

Not only are natural pet food and specific nutrients good for controlling epilepsy but so are disease-fighting antioxidant vitamins such as C and E, which can help protect your pet's immune system. Many holistic practitioners emphasize immune-strengthening vitamin C, which assists in detoxifying the body. And vitamin E, like fat, helps decrease inflammation of the brain, notes Dr. Scanlan. "A seizure is nothing more than an inflammatory process in the brain and nervous system. The strength or weakness of the immune system determines the severity of the resulting symptom. For example, a mild inflammatory process in the nervous system could trigger a headache while a major one could cause a seizure," says Dr. Goldstein.

Case in point: Katie is a six-year-old Irish setter who was having several multiple grand mal seizures a day. Phenobarbital and potassium bromide didn't appear to be alleviating her convulsions. Katie's veterinarian combined acupuncture treatments and vitamin E, which helped stabilize the dog. After the combo-therapy, the Irish setter's seizures stopped.

"In my experience, animals who are on a good vitamin and mineral program don't seem to suffer seizures," says holistic veterinarian Wendell O. Belfield. "Whenever an animal suffering from seizures is brought into my office, I ask the owner if the dog has been on supplements of any kind, and invariably the answer is no." Consult with your veterinarian to determine the type and dosage of multiple mineral and vitamin supplements that is best for your dog or cat.

REMEDY #5
VITAMIN B_6

Other essential vitamins can help stave off epilepsy as well. Dr. Belfield states, "It has long been known that a deficiency of vitamin B_6 or any interference with its function can cause seizures in any mammalian species, including man and dog." In fact, a lack of B_6 seems to be a common feature in many seizure situations, according to holistic vets.

Niacinamide, one of the common forms of B_6, may also be beneficial in combating epilepsy. One woman had a poodle who was having convulsive seizures. "She started to give the animal 25 mg of niacinamide, and in a week or so the attacks stopped," recalls Dr. Belfield.

Holistic vets maintain that the B vitamins are very important to nerve tissue. Use any natural B complex vitamin found at a health food store. (Consult with your veterinarian to determine the recommended daily allowance.)

REMEDY #6
HERBOLOGY

Herbal medicine derived from Mother Nature's plants can strengthen the nervous system and enhance the therapeutic diet. Historically, herbology has been used longer than any other form of medicine. Holistic experts swear by the antioxidant and chemical powers of these natural wonder drugs.

To control epilepsy, herbalists pay special attention to three herbs: valerian, skullcap, and oatstraw, according to Gregory L. Tilford, herbalist and CEO of Animals' Apawthecary (a company that manufactures low-alcohol herb extracts for dogs and cats) in Conner, Montana.

Tilford explains why these herbs play such an important role.

Valerian has been found to have a safe, sedative effect on the higher brain centers, which means it may play a role as an anticonvulsive in epileptic people and animals.

Skullcap works by reducing the nervous tension and nerve-related pain that is often associated with seizures and convulsions.

Oatstraw nourishes the entire nervous system and improves brain and nerve function, while acting as a mild sedative. This herb works well in cases of postadrenaline anxiety, which occurs after a convulsive seizure. This, in turn, makes oatstraw a useful long-term tonic for the epileptic, and it works well with skullcap and valerian.

Another multiple herbal remedy that holistic vets recommend is Tranquil complex made by Professional Health Products; it is available at health food stores.

REMEDY #7
HOMEOPATHY

Homeopathic remedies work on the premise of "like cures like," and they contain very small amounts of substances that would cause similar symptoms a patient is enduring if the substances were given to a healthy animal. "With epilepsy you often don't know what's causing the pet's seizures, so there's no single homeopathic prescription," says Dr. Blake, who incorporates homeopathic remedies for his patients. "Success occurs when you find a homeopathic remedy that fits the uniqueness of a single pet's symptoms."

For instance, a twelve-year-old poodle named Daisy was having countless petit mal seizures daily. Phenobarbital didn't offer relief, so Dr. Blake treated the epileptic canine with the homeopathic remedy silicea. After about three months on the remedy, Daisy no longer needed the phenobarbital.

"I have had great success using homeopathics to treat animals. They respond quickly to the right remedy, and homeopathics don't cause unpleasant side effects like drugs do," says Dr. Goldstein.

As an alternative to herbs, there are various homeopathic remedies that are quite useful in treating epilepsy when taken orally. Following are a few of Dr. Pitcairn's suggestions. Work with your veterinarian to get the correct dosage based on your pet's weight.

Thuja occidentalis 30C (arborvitae): Begin this once-a-month treatment, observe for a month, and if the problem is not better, try silicea (if the animal improves, discontinue the remedy but continue with the nutrition and other alternative methods already discussed).

Silicea 30C (silicon dioxide): Treat and observe for one month. If there is improvement, further treatment will not be needed.

Arnica montana 30C (mountain daisy): This remedy is indicated for the animal who has developed seizures after a head injury.

Tissue salts: According to Dr. Pitcairn, tissue salts can be used if the above treatments fail. They can be found in many health food stores and shouldn't be used in conjunction with other homeopathic medicines. Consider the following once-a-day tissue salt treatments for your pet's symptoms.

Tissue salt kali phosphoricum 6X (potassium phosphate) helps with nervous disturbances such as insomnia, irritability, or excessive nervousness by strengthening the nervous system. Tissue salt ferrum phosphoricum 6X (iron phosphate) is beneficial for seizures accompanied by head congestion. Tissue salt natrum sulphuricum 6X (sodium sulfate) should be administered if the epilepsy started after an injury to the head. Tissue salt silicea 6X (silicon dioxide) is useful for a seizure that occurs during sleep or at night.

For more detailed information, consult with your vet

or contact the International Association for Veterinary Homeopathy, 334 Knollwood Lane., Woodstock, GA 30188; (404) 516-5954.

CHAPTER 3

What You Can Do at Home

Antiseizure remedies do not stop with acupuncture and good nourishment for a dog's or a cat's body. There are preventive measures you can do at home that can help control seizures too. You can keep your pet seizure-free by creating a healthier world both indoors and outdoors. Holistic veterinary experts offer this at-home advice: lessen stress, get rid of toxins, and exercise your pet.

LESSEN STRESS

Some psychological, physical, and emotional factors, such as a visit the veterinarian, excessively itchy skin, or a new baby or dog, can wreak havoc on a dog or cat with epilepsy. What's more, a change in a pet's daily routine, such as traveling, may bring on sleep deprivation, which has triggered seizures in humans, according to research. An onset of seizures can also happen for no apparent reason.

"Try to decrease novelty, which can rev up stress levels," says John C. Wright, Ph.D., an animal behaviorist in Atlanta, Georgia. Pets thrive on consistency, so even if your own schedule is topsy-turvy, try to keep your epileptic pet's mealtimes and exercise times the same to provide a tranquil structure.

If an epileptic dog suffers from separation anxiety, the ritual of leaving your home (getting dressed, turning off the lights, jingling your keys) can add to stress levels. "If you're going out, don't make it a ritual display that makes it obvious you will be leaving, which adds to the dog's stress," says Dr. Wright. Leave abruptly, lessening the number of habitual tasks you usually perform before leaving, or use a different door. In most cases, this reduces your dog's arousal or anxiety. In turn, the situation stays calm and keeps your dog under control and less likely to suffer a stress-related seizure.

Before a seizure occurs, fear can play a strong role in an animal's behavior. Often, a dog runs to her owner in a state of fright, which only encourages the oncoming epileptic attack. Keeping calm and speaking softly to the animal can help soothe her. For epileptic cases in which emotions play a strong role, calming flower remedies (developed by Dr. Bach) found at health food stores can "alleviate stress and fear, which can reduce the odds of having a seizure," Dr. Blake says.

GET RID OF TOXINS

Like herbs, a clean and chemical-free environment can help protect your pet from toxins that may irritate the brain tissue, according to Dr. Pitcairn. That means keeping your pet away from cigarette smoke, car exhaust, chemicals (unnatural flea sprays, dips, and collars), a color TV, or an operating microwave oven—all of which affect the nervous system.

Many veterinarians believe that epilepsy stems from or is aggravated by yearly vaccinations. "It is triggered by allergic encephalitis, an ongoing, low-grade inflammation of the brain caused by a reaction to proteins and organisms in the vaccine," explains Dr. Pitcairn.

For starters, stay clear of chemical flea products. Instead, seek alternative, natural ways to control fleas, and use herbal formulas to repel fleas, ticks, and mosquitoes.

In addition, "Don't fret about the vaccinations that you've already given your dog or cat. As unbelievable as it sounds, homeopathy can counteract the undesired after-effects of vaccines, even for injections given years ago. The remedy *Thuja occidentalis* works even if your animal isn't sick right now," says Dr. Goldstein.

EXERCISE YOUR PET

Getting physical—whether it's running, swimming, or walking—isn't a cure-all for epilepsy; however, seizures may become less frequent. Why? Simply put, "regular physical activity can use up nervous energy," says Dr. Pitcairn, "just like sedatives can calm the nervous system down." Exercise also helps keep the animal fit and healthy.

Studies show that people who get physical exercise on a regular basis are less prone to illness and disease because exercise strengthens the immune system. Epileptic dogs and cats may reap health benefits from exercise, too. Brittany spaniel Dylan is naturally tranquil after running. His owner is thankful that exercise has helped control his epilepsy. Your dog should get at least twenty minutes of exercise each day. Unfortunately, 75 percent of pet dogs don't get enough of this health booster.

Cats need physical activity as well. Most cats enjoy playing with cat toys, which can strengthen the heart and lungs, improve body and muscle tone, keep a pet unstressed, and boost her well-being.

And be sure that your pet gets adequate water (distilled or filtered water is best) before and after exercise for total health.

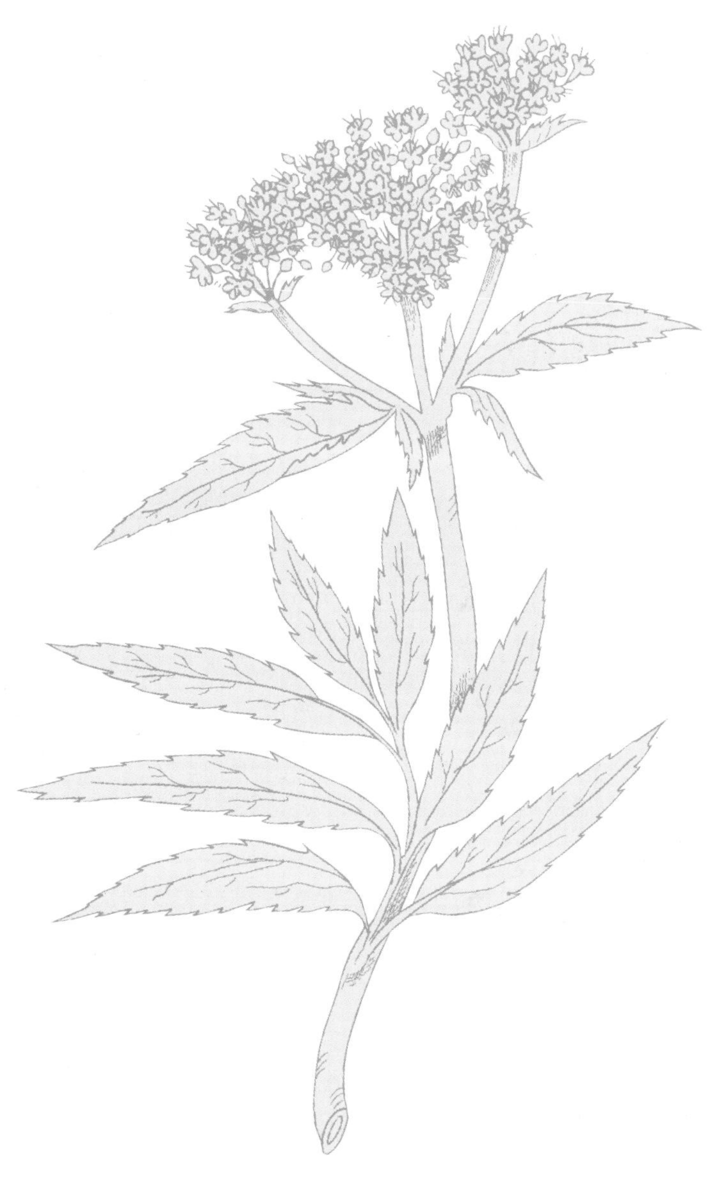

New advances

At the dawn of a new millennium, the number one treatment for epileptic pets is still conventional medicine, or drug therapy. The good news is that using medications in combination with alternative therapies is becoming more common, especially in difficult cases. Better still, in less-severe epileptic pets, holistic medicine is working oftentimes without any drugs at all.

Use of conventional drugs does have some positive aspects, though. "As long as allopathic—or conventional—medicine is the predominant treatment, vets and pet owners will give pets drugs,

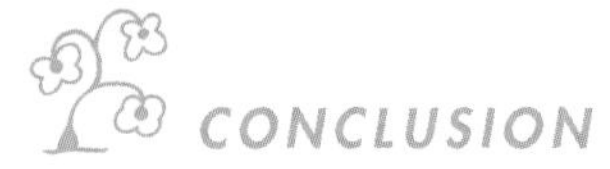

and pharmaceutical companies will create new and improved drugs," says holistic practitioner Charles Loops, D.V.M., in Pittsboro, North Carolina. Currently, for instance, scientists at Ohio State University are researching a new anticonvulsant drug therapy for cats that combines phenobarbital and potassium bromide with Tranxene, which is a tranquilizer.

But times are changing. "I treat a lot of epilepsy where the owners have not used any drugs. There are people who will immediately seek out an alternative. They don't want to put their pets on barbiturates. Usually it's the people who treat their own bodies holistically," adds Dr. Loops.

Sometimes, trying new superalternative strategies is best, even if it means turning to experimental antiseizure treatments that humans resort to, such as the ketogenic diet. Today, humans and pet owners are seeking this diet as an alternative to drug therapy for controlling seizures. Primarily used on children, this program is difficult to follow, and it is controversial in both the conventional and holistic medicine worlds.

A few of Dr. Loops's clients, in fact, have inquired about the antiseizure, high-fat k-diet, and one enthusiastic individual sent him a copy of the book *The Epilepsy Diet Treatment: An Introduction to the Ketogenic Diet*. Some holistic vets, such as Dr. Scanlan, prescribe the k-diet to some of their epileptic patients. Scanlan has had impressive results with the diet combined with acupuncture.

"When a body uses fat as its basic fuel instead of carbohydrates or protein, ketone bodies are formed—hence the name ketogenic diet. The k-diet limits the amount of protein to only what is needed by the body, decreases carbohydrate levels to as close to zero as possible, and increases the amount of fat," explains Dr. Scanlan. "One way to do this is to add fat or oil to the diet, depending on the size of the animal. When doing this, be sure to add vitamin E, lecithin, and choline, and decrease the regular food by half. If your pet is still hungry, he can have apples or vegetables as a treat, or high-fat potato chips," she adds.

Sample Homemade K-Diet Meal Plan

Amounts given are for one meal.

	35-lb Dog	**10-lb Dog**
*Ground chicken**	*½ cup*	*¼ cup*
Ground carrots	*¼ cup*	*2 Tbs*
Ground broccoli	*¼ cup*	*2 Tbs*
Canola oil	*3 oz*	*1 ½ Tbs*
Vitamin E	*200 IU*	*100 IU*
Calcium	*500 mg*	*200 mg*
Kelp powder	*small pinch*	*sprinkle*
Cholodin (a high-choline B vitamin tablet)	*1 tablet*	*¼ tablet*
Lecithin granules	*small pinch*	*sprinkle*

Mix all the ingredients together. Serve two meals a day.

**Many holistic veterinarians feel that raw meat is preferable to cooked. Raw meat has some healthy properties that cooked meat does not have; however, raw ground meat is also more likely to contain* E. coli *and* Salmonella. *(Poultry is especially prone to containing* Salmonella.*) The longer that ground meat sits around (even refrigerated), the more likely it is to contain unwanted bacteria. To minimize the threat of severe disease, be sure that the meat you feed your pet is ground fresh just before you buy it and that you use it within a few days of purchase. If you feel uncomfortable serving raw meat to your pet, you can cook the meat before serving it.*

Guidelines for the k-diet are as follows:

- This diet should not be used by any animal who is overweight or who has had pancreatitis.
- Cats probably should not be put on this diet because it tends to add pounds, and overweight cats have problems with diabetes and potentially fatal liver problems.
- Any change to this diet should be gradual, over a ten-day period.
- For the first three days, ¼ of the diet should be the k-diet, with ¾ of the old diet.
- For the next three days, the pet should eat ½ k-diet and ½ old diet.

For the next three days, feed your pet ¾ k-diet and ¼ old diet.

 Finally, feed him 100 percent k-diet.

Use ground meat or poultry, mixed half-and-half with ground vegetables (raw or steamed carrots, broccoli, or dark-green/leafy vegetables).

 Don't forget vitamin and mineral supplements.

INTERNET MEDICAL ADVICE

Unlike TV, the Internet can connect you with other people in similar situations. "People can be more useful," says Tom Ferguson, M.D., author of *Health Online*, a book about finding health data electronically.

Often owners of epileptic pets start out by looking for disease information (for example, using the key words "canine seizures"), and wind up using the Internet to stay in touch with other pet owners experiencing the same dilemma. Through "chat rooms" and online discussion groups, you can find new information and support.

Studies and articles provided by writers, veterinarians, and pet experts at universities are available to the

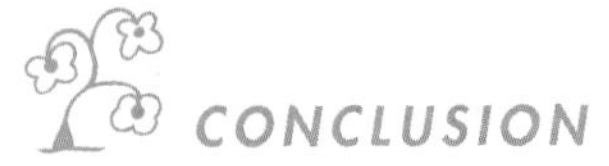

public online. Web sites list sources of information. Be wary, however. Sometimes information is not current, so check the date that the data was posted and see if it has been updated.

Canine Epilepsy Online Resources:

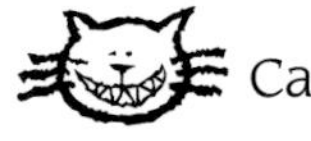 Canine Epilepsy Web Site:
www.world.std.com/~tolenio/epilepsy.html

Alternative veterinary medicine Web site:
www.altvetmed.com

Epil-K9: an Internet canine epilepsy mailing list. To subscribe to Epil-K9, send E-mail to:

LISTSERV@APPLE.EASE.LSOFT.COM
Leave the subject blank. In the body, type:
subscribe Epil-K9 (your name)

There is a canine epilepsy chat on the Internet at 12 P.M. and 8 P.M., EST. Dalnet is the server. Consult the Canine Epilepsy Web Site (above) for the server addresses and ports. Visit www.dalnet.com for help.

Yahoo is a good search engine to find information on epilepsy. Go to www.yahoo.com and search for "seizures and epilepsy" for all information, or search "canine seizures" or "canine epilepsy" to restrict information to dogs.

Send E-mail to ACVM@aol.com for a listing of all the vet neurologists in the U.S.

The Merck Manual, which is for people but much of the information translates to dogs, has information on epilepsy: www.merck.com. Then click on the button that says "Publications: Merck Manual."

There are a number of human epilepsy bulletin boards and resources that some pet owners also find useful. They're listed at:

www.neuro.wustl.edu/epilepsy/index.html.

FAITH HEALING

New studies are showing that faith, prayer, and religious practices may be another holistic-welcome prescription for any illness. In fact, The National Institutes of Health has found spirituality is healing for every condition from heart disease to age-related problems.

One cat owner believes the healing power of faith may help control epilepsy, too. No sooner than

Tom Davis adopted an abandoned young Russian blue feline, Lucky, did trouble begin. Lucky began having "spooky" grand mal seizures almost every other day. Phenobarbital helped, but Lucky's guardian went one step further: A one-hour, hands-on, faith-healing session with a spiritual guide and his cat, and two weeks later things changed. Lucky now suffers only two petit mal seizures a month. She is still on medication but is much more playful and is grooming herself, too, reports Davis. Like Tom, more and more cat and dog owners are beating their pets' seizures by incorporating alternative therapies used to control epilepsy with medications.

SAFETY PRECAUTIONS

Laura Larsen who owns Tuff Guy, a cocker spaniel, recalls her dog's first seizure. And for her dog's sake, she kept her cool. "I had seen them before in humans, so I knew I needed to stay near him so he couldn't hurt himself. He knew I was there the whole time as far as I could tell," she says.

All epileptic pet owners need to decrease their pets' chances of hurting themselves during a seizure. These hints can help your cat or dog stay clear of many potential hazards:

- Stay calm during a seizure and talk to your pet in a soothing voice.

- Keep your pet on the floor and away from any objects. Do not allow him to fall off furniture or down stairs.

- To prevent choking, remove his collar and leash. Keep your hands away from his mouth. Your pet is not aggressive during a seizure, but he has no control of his jaw muscles and may bite anything put into his mouth.

- Dogs cannot swallow their tongues. Do not try to muzzle your pet, give him any medication, or manually restrain the tongue during a fit.

- Be aware that your pet may pass stool or urine during or after a seizure.

- Most seizures last less than sixty seconds and are not life threatening; however, if your pet has repeated seizures for more than five minutes or fails to regain consciousness between seizures, contact your vet immediately.

- Keep a journal of the seizures, describing the date, time, duration, and severity of each seizure.

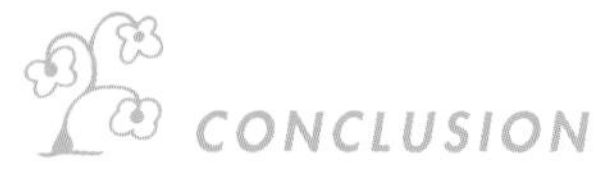

Here are more savvy tips from the experts:

Follow your vet's instructions. Do not stop or change medication or dosages without a consultation. Abruptly stopping medication can result in a cluster of seizures.

Be patient and willing to try another form of treatment.

If your breed club sponsors a health registry or research project on seizures or epilepsy, please join. Hopefully, studies on epilepsy will help us discover how epilepsy is inherited and help us find a genetic (or diagnostic) test such as the ones we have for hip dysplasia and other pet diseases. This will help breeders breed selectively and control the epilepsy epidemic.

If your pet is diagnosed with epilepsy, seek a second opinion for your pet's body and your peace of mind.

YOU CAN'T ARGUE WITH SUCCESS

Plenty of pets are reaping the benefits of holistic medicine. Take a look at three success stories:

Eric, a thin, dignified ten-year-old German short-haired pointer fell victim to a brain tumor, which caused seizures. At first his seizures were controlled by phenobarbital because the brain tumor was too deep to be removed safely. As his tumor continued to grow, Eric's seizures became difficult to control. Even with increased levels of phenobarbital combined with potassium bromide, Eric's seizures didn't stop. Eric's vet and owner treated his epilepsy with acupuncture and a ketogenic diet, teamed with his original medication, and were able to control Eric's seizures. The dog was able to live another year before his seizures became too difficult to control.

Ramona, a slim, bubbly, white five-and-a half-year-old shepherd mixed breed suffered cluster seizures that were only partially controlled by phenobarbital and potassium bromide. She still had at least three seizures a month, usually in a cluster. With acupuncture and a ketogenic diet, Ramona became seizure-free.

Susie, a solemn two-and-a-half-year-old mixed breed, had her seizures controlled by phenobarbital and potassium bromide, but the medications made her sleep all the time. Her owner was determined to take her off all medication. Her owner fed her a ketogenic diet, which allowed Susie's medication to be decreased. Susie slept much less and started playing like a puppy.

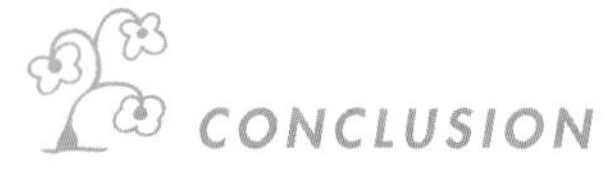

CONCLUSION

Although many epileptic pets improve with holistic remedies, there remain an estimated 20 to 30 percent of epileptic pets whose conditions will never be controlled. Epilepsy should not shorten an affected pet's life span, though, unless the animal's seizures are extremely frequent or they continue despite therapy.

Dylan is another one of the lucky ones. Since undergoing alternative treatments—including antioxidant-rich pet food, exercise, and a chemical-free lifestyle—he has been almost seizure-free without taking anticonvulsant medication.

Before starting a treatment plan, bear in mind that you should discuss all the options with your veterinarian. Countless epileptic pets are living happy and healthy lives, thanks to holistic remedies.

For more information on holistic medicine or to find out how you can consult a holistic veterinarian in your area, contact: American Holistic Veterinary Medical Association, 2214 Old Emmorton Rd., Bel Air, MD 21015; (410) 569-0795.

SELECTED BIBLIOGRAPHY

Much of the research and information on natural medicine comes from a variety of sources that can be difficult to find. While the amount of written research is growing, a lot of the information still can only be found in unpublished sources. In addition to using the conventional sources such as books, magazines, and veterinary journals, the author interviewed holistic and conventional veterinarians and researched several unpublished sources including news releases and articles from the Internet. Following are sources in which you can find more information on epilepsy.

Books and Magazines

Belfield, O. Wendell and Zucker, Martin. *How to Have a Healthier Dog: The Benefits of Vitamins and Minerals for Your Dog's Life Cycles*. A Signet Book, 1981.

Ferguson, Tom, M.D. *Health Online*. Addison-Wesley, 1995.

Freeman, John. *The Epilepsy Diet Treatment: An Introduction to the Ketogenic Diet*. Demo Vermande, 1996.

Pitcairn, Richard H., D.V.M., Ph.D., and Susan Hubble Pitcarin. *Dr. Pitcairn's Complete Guide to Natural Health for Dogs and Cats*. Emmaus, PA: Rodale, 1995.

Plechner J. Alfred, D.V.M., and Martin Zucker. *Pet Allergies: Remedies for an Epidemic*. Los Angeles: J.P. Enterprises, 1986.

Seizures and Epilepsy in Dogs. Brillig Hill, Inc., Veterinary Practice Publishing Co. 1993. Ask your veterinarian to order this brochure by writing to Veterinary Practice Publishing Company, P.O. Box 6050, Mission Viejo, CA 92690.

Shojai, Amy D. *The Purina Encyclopedia of Cat Care.* New York: Ballantine Books, 1998.

Internet and Other Sources

Goldstein, Bob, V.M.D., and Susan Goldstein. *Healing and Preventing the Fourteen Most Dangerous Pet Diseases.* Pamphlet.

Goldstein, Bob, V.M.D., and Susan Goldstein. *Love of Animals* newsletter. To subscribe to the *Love of Animals* newsletter or to receive volumes, pamphlets, and other pet-related information from Dr. Bob Goldstein and Susan Goldstein, call Earth Animals at 1-800-211-6365.

Wiersma-Aylward, Alicia. *Canine Epilepsy.* (http://www.k9web.com/dog-faqs/medical/epilepsy.html) Copyright 1995.

ABOUT THE AUTHOR

Cal Orey, a freelance writer based in northern California, has a master's degree in English from San Francisco State University. In the past decade, she has written hundreds of articles about human and pet health in many national magazines, including *Dog Fancy* and *Natural Dog.* She owns a nine-year-old Brittany spaniel, Dylan, and a look-alike thirteen-year-old laid-back cat named Alex. The author is thankful for the holistic remedies that have helped control Dylan's epilepsy.

ABOUT THE VETERINARIAN

Dr. Nancy Scanlan graduated from the University of California, Davis, in 1970. She has used nutritional therapy since her senior year there. She has been certified in veterinary acupuncture since 1988 and has taught animal health and animal science for ten years. Dr. Scanlan regularly writes articles for various pet-related magazines. She currently practices holistic-only medicine in California, using acupuncture, nutritional therapy, Chinese and Western herbs, trigger point therapy, and Chiropractic. If you are interested in getting in touch with Dr. Scanlan, contact the American Holistic Veterinary Medical Association.

For more about natural pet care, look for *Natural Cat* and *Natural Dog* magazines at pet stores and selected newsstands.

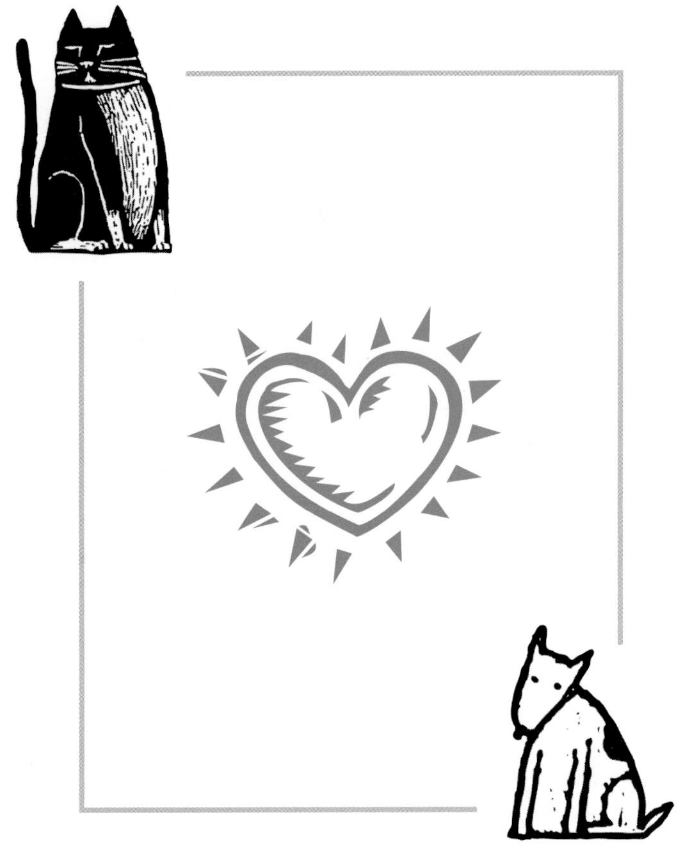